REVIEWS

The UCLA BrainSPORT Program and the CDC have partnered with USA Football and the NFL to help reduce sport-related brain injuries, especially those involving concussions in youth sports. Our collective goal is to help inform and educate sports-related organizations and their coaches, players, and parents about the need to provide a safe and positive playing and learning environment for all participants. It is clear that this is also the primary objective of Concussion Awareness *by Mike Shaw. The book offers great insights into concussions, how to identify them, aftercare, and return to play. This information is essential for anyone involved with sports and coaching, at any level.*

—Constance Johnson
  UCLA BrainSPORT Program Director

As the father of professional athletes in baseball and football, I heartily endorse this new handbook Concussion Awareness. *I appreciate the emphasis on safety awareness for all athletes, and especially the focus on youth sports. Combating the threat of concussions and the long term problems they can cause is a goal I share whole-heartedly. I am delighted that Mathnasium supports the publication of this much-needed volume.*

—Jeff Pudewell, Mathnasium Franchise, California
  www.mathnasium.com

Watering Seeds Organization is a non-profit organization that creates sports and recreational opportunities for wounded warriors and physically challenged individuals. WSO provides education, training, and the rehabilitation necessary to help get individuals, "off the sidelines and into the game." We work with schools, cities, and other foundations nationwide on the very important work of informing and educating sports-related organizations and their coaches, players, and parents about the need to provide a safe and positive playing and learning environment for all participants. After reading Concussion Awareness, *it was obvious to us that the goal of the author was to write a resource guide for coaches, players, and parents to follow in providing that safe and positive playing and learning environment. We would like to congratulate you. You have succeeded. We will be recommending the book at all our events and programs. We know it will be very helpful to all concerned.*

—Brady Mazzola, Founder, Watering Seeds Organization
  www.wateringseeds.org

REVIEWS

I have been officiating high school football and baseball for the last 22 years, and college lacrosse for the last 8 years. I've seen many injuries that I feel could have been avoided if more emphasis had been placed on helping coaches, parents, and administrators protect their players. Everybody involved in sports, including doctors, should read the book Concussion Awareness, which focuses on awareness of what can and should be done to protect players. I can tell you that rules are also being updated and changed to protect the players. The NFL is setting a good example with its rule requiring players to get clearance from a doctor before returning to play. .

—Bernard Battle, BBonKeys@gmail.com;
   High School Sports Officiating San Diego

Over the last 5 years I have had the honor of producing the — Celebrate America Tour — featuring one of the top motivational speakers in the country, Bob "Mr. Inspiration" Wieland. Mr. Wieland has one of the top ranked high school assembly programs in America. In communities everywhere, parents, students, coaches and teachers are trying to navigate many challenges: cyber bullying, distracted driving, drugs, alcohol, performing under pressure, and just trying to fit in. In the sports world, the trending challenge is concussion related. I want to encourage everyone to add the book Concussion Awareness, to you game plan for success. You will be glad you did!

—Brett Bohl, Executive Producer / Founder
   Celebrate America Tour — featuring Bob Wieland
   www.bobwieland.com

Having been a participant in martial arts and combative sports for over fifty years I am pleased that a group of informed individuals are focusing attention on concussions and the attendant damage that often follows. I have had concerns about young athletes and the long term effects of head injuries as they reach maturity and advancing age. Bravo for shining a light that will keep us safer after our competing days are past.

—Professor Bob Kent, Chow Hoon Goshinjutsu 7th degree, Judo 5th degree,
   Golden Gloves Boxing and AAU Boxing

REVIEWS

I just finished reading Concussion Awareness *by Coach Shaw, and it is awesome. The book offers great insights into concussions, how to identify them, aftercare, and return to play. This information is essential for anyone coaching or training youngsters in football or other sports. Better understanding of what concussions are and how to deal with them—both on the field and afterward—is essential. I appreciated the way Coach Shaw presented the concerns of many parents and others, and I also appreciated the values he emphasized and stressed: things like character, teamwork, leadership, sportsmanship, and ethics. I learned all these things from Coach Shaw, and I feel that it helped me build a firm and solid foundation. As I am now coaching my son and his youth team, I strive to give them a similar experience and teach the same values that were drilled into me. Thank you for being such an amazing coach and, more importantly, for being such a great role model, father figure, and man.*

—Daylon McCutcheon
 former USC Trojan and Cleveland Browns cornerback

We have certainly come a long way in our understanding of how blows to the head can harm the brain. Together with continued research, education, open dialogue, and books like Concussion Awareness *by Mike Shaw, we can help reduce the flow of misinformation and fear that can lead to parents pulling their kids out of competitive sports. Doing so would deprive generations to come of the sense of accomplishment, thrill of competition, and camaraderie that go hand in hand with sports. I truly believe the person I am today is due, in large part, to having played competitive sports beginning in kindergarten. In hindsight, I may not have returned to practice so quickly after what I can now see were clearly concussions; however, I certainly would have still chosen to play competitive sports, even with this new knowledge and understanding. Missing out on the competition, accomplishments, memories, and relationships that were gained would be much scarier than any possible injury. This book is a must-read for anyone involved with youth sports at any level.*

—Scott Catlin ,Facebook.com/Catlinmma; Twitter:@ScottCatlinMMA;
 high school, college, and arena football veteran; 6 year MMA career football and MMA coach; father of autistic son; B/A Sociology JD, Thomas Jefferson School of Law

ACKNOWLEDGEMENTS

I would like to thank a number of people for their considerable input in helping get this project up and running. First, I'd be remiss if I didn't give the highest accolades to my wife who not only allowed me to coach, but joined in as Athletic Director, League Treasurer and eventually President of the organization. We've been married for 45 years, and I'm unmerciful in my teasing her constantly, but she is amazingly able to defend herself with humor and dignity. The last couple of churches we have attended call her "Saint Toni" because she's been married to me for so long. I think that they are being overly judgmental in their assessment of me, but my wife says I bring it all on myself, so I guess it's true that I married UP. When I married her, I knew I married "Mrs. Right." I didn't know her first name was "Always!"

I must also thank the great coaches I have worked with over the years. In Rowland Heights, I had the distinct pleasure of working with Harry Robinson, one of the most honest and truly dedicated men I've ever had the privilege of knowing. With him, Craig Snyder, Rick Amontorp, Ralph Harris, and more.

More recently, I coached at Oaks Christian School under Bill Ridell, a Hall of Fame player AND coach, who has forgotten more about coaching than I could ever learn. His leadership and integrity is the primary reason the football program has been so successful. Also, at Oaks, the finest coach I've ever met is Clay Matthews, 19 years in the NFL, and the Defensive Coordinator par excellence. Bob Richards was the primary offensive and defensive line coach. The Offensive Coordinator/part time genius was Mark Bates. Mike Maio was the special teams guru and these guys were the most amazing coaches I've ever seen on one staff.

At the youth level, my wife and I have made friendships that are lasting a lifetime. The parents and families of the boys I had the distinct honor to coach have become as close as any family could ever hope.

I would be remiss if I didn't acknowledge Orange County Jr. All American Football. There are many people there with whom I find myself so deeply indebted because of their support, friendship and dedication to youth football. This organization for the last couple of decades has been headed up by Bob Barna, his wife Suzie and a great board of directors, chapter presidents and all their staffs and of course the coaches. All these youth organizations who so painstakingly pour themselves into their avocation to serve our young people are to be gratefully commended for their unpaid devotion.

Additionally, many people have encouraged me in writing this book. My partners in this enterprise include my Publisher, Bob Howland, President of Griffin Publishing, Vincent Jackson, Vice President of B3NET, Inc., website design and internet excellence and Keith Tetz, Director of Mathnasium. Also, Chad Fenwick of the Los Angeles Unified School District for his insights and suggestions. And thank-you to all the good people at Mind Over Media, Inc. for their assistance throughout the development of this project.

But most of all, I thank the Lord for giving me the opportunity to get involved in the lives of so many amazing people.

The young people with whom I've had the honor of coaching gave me far more than I could ever give them. As coaches we teach the sport; we impart life lessons as well as football instruction; we love them, guide, and direct them; and at the youth level, we don't get paid, but by the end of the season, we have been OVER paid because these kids give us their hearts.

FORWARD
By Bill Redell, Head Coach, Oaks Christian High School

This is an important book not only because it informs the reader of the essential information concerning the consequences of a concussion, but it addresses much more, including the myths and facts of a concussion, and the protocols of returning the injured player to his or her sport or simply back to normal activities.

As a football coach and former professional football player, I believe this book should be part of the training materials necessary for all coaches, trainers, parents, administrators and medical professionals. As coaches, we are in the business of providing an educational and safe environment for athletes regardless of level, whether reaching the youth, high school, college or professional athletes. Parents are naturally concerned about the protection of their children. We must provide the proper equipment, playing field conditions and a coaching methodology which addresses safety, teamwork and positive life lessons.

This book is designed to help the reader understand what a concussion is, how to recognize it, and how to deal with it regardless of when or where it happens, both in and outside of the sports environment. One of the primary goals is to raise awareness of how easy it is to overlook the basic symptoms of a concussion, and that concussions are not limited to contact sports like football and ice hockey. They can include non-helmeted activities involving cheerleaders, soccer players, housewives, and car accident victims. The "On-field Guidelines Card" is an excellent resource for immediate assessment of a head, neck or spinal injury and trainers will view it as a vital tool in evaluating impact injuries. The book also covers protocols for dealing with concussions both on and off the playing field, and the return to normal activity considerations.

The section covering the myths and facts underscores the misunderstanding many people have concerning the concussion issue. The book also deals with the problem of overreaction by some parents and even medical personnel. It includes concussion research, new product development "Baseline Testing" concerns and how to determine the severity or grade of concussion.

I have known Mike Shaw for more than 20 years. Not only did he do an outstanding job on our coaching staff at Oaks Christian High School, Mike also conducted some of the finest coaching clinics I have ever seen. Mike's expertise goes beyond coaching to the areas of sports injuries, management of injuries and return to play for the athlete. It is a pleasure for me to recommend this book to all the coaches, trainers, parents and athletes. Everyone can derive something very positive from this presentation of concussion awareness.

Bill Redell, member of the College Football Hall of Fame as both a player and a coach. Head coach at Oaks Christian High School in Westlake Village, California. Went to USC on a scholarship, transferred to Occidental College. Named to the NAIA All-America team in 1963. Played six years in the Canadian Football League. Coached at Cal State University, Fullerton and Cal Lutheran University. At the high school level, Bill has won six CIF Championships.

©2015 by Mike Shaw

This publication is a creative work fully protected by all applicable rights. All rights reserved. No portion of this book may be reproduced or transmitted in any form or by any means, electronic or mechanical, including fax, photocopy, or recording, or any other information storage or retrieval system by anyone. This book may not be reproduced in its entirety without written permission of the author or publisher.

Co-Publisher, Concussion Awareness Institute LLC is an organization dedicated to providing information regarding the problems of injuries, primarily concussions. Much of this work is generally focused on sports but we note that many concussions come from simply living life. A fall down the stairs or sliding in the snow, an automobile accident, bumping into something, even the smallest of accidents can result in a concussion. This book is the first step in a series of explorations into the goal of removing the mystery of concussion, while future endeavors will deal with other injuries, prevention, reduction of such injuries, and cutting edge research compiled from a variety of resources. We will be sharing information with other foundations and research organizations who agree that the majority of injuries can be dramatically reduced through better equipment, rule changes which positively affect sports, certification of coach and trainers on concussion protocols and much more. Our website will be a dissemination hub of information delivering the latest and greatest research and development on reducing injuries in sports and in life. Please comment on the information presented herein by visiting our website at: **ConcussionAwarenessInstitute.com**

1-58000-138-6

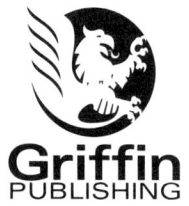

Griffin Publishing USA

Publisher: Robert M. Howland

bob@griffinpublishing.com

Copy Editor: RosAnne Tetz, Mind Over Media, Inc.

Manufactured in the United States of America

Printed by: Winbrook, Inc.

Book Design: m2design group, www.m2dg.com

Although the author and publisher have researched many sources to assure accuracy and completeness of the information in this book, we assume no responsibility whatsoever for errors, inaccuracies, omissions, or other inconsistencies herein. The purpose is to help educate the reader about concussions and role coaches, trainers, parents, and athletes play in dealing with concussions both on and off the playing field.

This book is in no way intended to be a substitute for the medical advice of a trusted medical professional. Any application of the advice herein is at the reader's own discretion and risk.

Also, in the interest of brevity, the author and publisher have chosen to use the standard English form of address. Pleased be advised that this usage is not meant to suggest a restriction to, nor an endorsement of, any individual or group of individuals, either by age, gender, or athletic ability. The author and publisher certainly acknowledge that boys and girls, men and women, of every age and physical condition are actively involved in sports, and we encourage everyone to enjoy the sports of his or her choice.

INTRODUCTION

Don't be so traumatized by the bad press, that you remove your child from a sport.

Okay, so what's the deal about concussions? Have they become so pervasive that parents shouldn't allow their kids to play sports such as football, hockey, baseball, lacrosse, wrestling, or even participate in cheerleading? It seems that parental concern has taken a turn towards overreaction rather than examination of the evidence. While not an attempt to practice medicine, much will be explained in this book about concussions. This book has been written for coaches, trainers, athletes, administrators, moms, dads, and sports fans of all kinds, using language and explanations that are both clear and understandable.

Again, do not be so traumatized by all the negative press on concussions that you decide to remove your child from participating in sports, and remember contact sports are not the problem. A CBS news report by Jan Crawford, really underscored the problem with overreaction regarding the concussion issues. As she and so many others have stated, the vast majority of concussions are mild and caution should certainly be exercised. But removing kids from certain sports deprives them of some of the greatest life lessons they will ever experience. The joys of competition, learning sportsmanship, the camaraderie, the fellowship, the lifelong friendships, the recognition for a job well done, all are part of playing youth sports. Parents and families are to be commended for their care, concern and involvement in the activities of their children, but also, to be cognizant of the need their youngster has to be encouraged by their family to positively participate with others in their own peer groups.

The vast majority of the time, an impact in sports or even in everyday life does NOT result in a concussion. However, it is far better to err on the side of caution than to tell the injured party, "Just walk it off," or "Hey, it's nothing, you'll be fine." Part of the accountability of a parent, coach, administrator, or trainer is to ALWAYS act in the best interest of those over whom we have responsibility.

One of the most important issues we must address in coaching is the need to understand the duty that accompanies the title. Winning the game is great, but regardless of the philosophies of many coaches—particularly at the youth, high school, and to some degree college level—winning is secondary to providing a safe and positive learning experience for your players.

TABLE OF CONTENTS

1 **REVIEWS**
3 **TITLE PAGE**
4 **ACKNOWLEDGEMENTS**
5 **FORWARD**
6 **COPYRIGHT PAGE**
7 **INTRODUCTION**
10 **CHAPTER 1:** What is a Concussion?
Recognizing a concussion
The brain's reaction to a concussion

11 **CHAPTER 2:** Signs and Symptoms of a Concussion
Cognitive: thought processes, memory
Physical
Emotional
Sleep issues

13 **CHAPTER 3:** Are There Different Grades of Severity of Concussions?
Grade 1
Grade 2
Grade 3

14 **CHAPTER 4:** What to Do if a Concussion Occurs

15 **CHAPTER 5:** Aftercare of a Concussion
Responsibilities of parents and family
Responsibilities of coaches and trainers
Responsibilities of medical professionals

17 **CHAPTER 6:** Professional's Protocols for Concussion Management
Physical limitations
Cognitive limitations
Testing

18 **CHAPTER 7:** When to Seek Medical Attention After Receiving a Head Injury

19 **CHAPTER 8:** Protocols for Returning to Play or Activity
Four steps
Scheduling recover
Observation

21 **CHAPTER 9:** **Concussion Myths and Facts**
Vital information

23 **CHAPTER 10:** **How Do We Prevent or Reduce the Occurrence of Concussions?**
Helmet issues
Non-helmet sports
Cheerleading

26 **CHAPTER 11:** **Can We Prevent Concussions From Ever Happening?**
No—but we can reduce the instances of concussion
Know your coach
Know the rules of the game
Get involved with the organization in a positive way

28 **CHAPTER 12:** **On-Field Assessment Guide (The Card)**
Comprehensive on-field assessment card for coaches and trainers
The do's and don'ts of on-field assessment
Certification availabilities

30 **CHAPTER 13:** **What is Being Done to Research the Long- and Short-Term Issues and Damages Caused by Concussions?**

31 **CHAPTER 14:** **A Word to Coaches**
Things have changed
Coaching ethics
Coaching philosophy
Objectives

34 **CHAPTER 15:** **What is the Issue of "Baseline Testing?"**
Why?
Who does it?
What is the cost?

35 **CHAPTER 16:** **Case Studies**

37 **CHAPTER 17:** **Fundraising**

39 **ADVERTISEMENTS**

40 **SPONSORS**

Most concussions occur without a loss of consciousness.

CHAPTER 1:
What is a Concussion?

A concussion is typically the result of trauma to the brain, often caused by a direct blow to the head or even an indirect blow to the body. Furthermore, a concussion is often characterized as an injury to the brain in which symptoms resolve of their own accord.

How do we recognize a concussion?

These symptoms usually reflect an operational issue to the brain and may include headaches, nausea, difficulty with conscious intellectual activity (thinking, reasoning, remembering, and concentrating) or emotional reactivity (irritability, moodiness, sadness), and continued sleep disturbances, or changes in appetite or energy levels. A concussion is considered a brain injury. You do not need to be "knocked out" for a concussion to occur; in fact, most concussions occur without a loss of consciousness. If you have had your "bell rung," it is most likely that you have had a concussion.

What happens to the brain during a concussion?

The adult brain is an organ that weighs about three pounds and is more or less floating inside the skull. It is suspended in cerebral spinal fluid, which acts as a shock absorber for minor impacts. When the brain is forced to move rapidly inside the skull, a concussion is often the result. A direct blow to the head or an impact that causes a whiplash effect to the body can create the concussion. The impact rapidly accelerates the head, and the brain strikes the inner skull. When the head decelerates and stops its motion (whiplash), the brain then collides with the opposite side of the inner skull. Additionally, a rotational concussion can occur, in which the head rapidly rotates from one side to another causing shearing and straining of brain tissues. In either case, delicate neural pathways in the brain can become damaged causing sensory or neurological issues.

CHAPTER 2: Signs and Symptoms of a Concussion

Concussion symptoms do not necessarily present themselves immediately.

What are some of the signs of a concussion?
Many of the symptoms are not necessarily going to present themselves immediately. The following are usually early onset symptoms and will be explained in greater detail in the next chapter.

Early Signs:
- Confused about assignment or position
- Appears dazed or disoriented
- Doesn't remember what happened before the impact event
- Doesn't remember what happened after the impact event
- Is unsure of game, score, or opponent
- Moves clumsily
- Responds to questions slowly or not at all
- Loses consciousness (even briefly)
- Shows unusual behavior or personality change

Symptoms of a concussion range from mild to severe and can last for hours, days, weeks, or even months. If you notice any symptoms of a concussion, contact your doctor. Symptoms of a concussion fit into four main categories:

Cognitive: Thought processes and memory
- Inability to remember or think clearly. Examples would include not knowing the day or time, where they are, or what they were engaged in at the time of the injury. Short-term memory loss is a certain indication of concussion. For example, the victim may ask, "Who won the game?" Response: "We did." Then, "What was the score?" Response: "21 to 14." Then he may ask again, "Great, who won the game?"
- Concentration impairment, including the inability to focus on even simple things and ideas. It can also manifest as the incapacity to follow instructions or respond intelligently to any new information or ideas.
- The injured party may express the feeling that everything is slowing down. Sometimes a degree of mild panic may set in or even uncontrollable laughter or weeping. When asked why, their response is often, "I don't know."

Physical
- One of the first indications of a concussion is often a mild or severe headache. The injured person often exhibits a painful response or sensitivity to light. Even sensory input such as noise or several people talking to the injured individual at the same time can trigger mild to extreme discomfort.

- If possible, it is important to discern any kind of visual impairment. Check the eyes for dilation. If the pupils do not respond to light, it is more than likely a concussion. If the injured person complains of blurry vision or extreme visual loss, especially if he has received a blow to the head, get a doctor involved as soon as possible. Try not to move the person until a doctor or medical professional has an opportunity to assess and diagnose the problem.
- Another symptom can be nausea or vomiting. Often, this issue will not manifest itself until the player or injured person has been up and moving around for a while.
- Having little or no energy can also be an indication of a concussion.
- Balance can be affected either mildly or radically depending on the severity of the concussion. When injured people have difficulty sitting up, raising their arms, or walking, or if they display any other new physical limitation, they should be monitored closely.

Emotional

- Mood can be an indicator of concussion. Mood swings from elation to depression can appear suddenly or more slowly, depending on the extent and severity of the concussion.
- The injured person may become easily upset over seemingly unimportant or inconsequential issues.
- Anxiety or abnormal nervousness.
- Emotions are important when checking for any kind of head injury. If the injured person is displaying more or deeper emotional behavior than normal, continue to observe the individual. These symptoms usually abate fairly quickly, but paying close attention is advised.

Sleep issues

- Difficulty falling asleep.
- Sleeping more than normal.
- Sleeping less than normal.
- Nightmares, as well as tossing and turning more than usual.
- The issues with sleep may sound confusing, but the main thing is to be cautious and aware of anything that is out of the norm.

Although children exhibit the same indications of a concussion as an adult, there are some additional issues that a parent must consider when it comes to their child. The following are a few of those indicators:

- Sustained headache, one about which the child continues to complain.
- Dietary changes. With babies, the mother may notice that the child is not nursing the way he or she normally does. With young children, their eating habits may change a little or a lot.
- The way children play may be affected. Even their enthusiasm or lack thereof may indicate that a problem exists.
- Loss of interest in activities they once enjoyed, such as toys, games, or events they once looked forward to.
- Throwing tantrums or getting angry more quickly and/or more often than normal.
- Very young children may lose their balance more easily or lose control of recently acquired skills such as walking, toilet training, etc.
- Persistent sadness.
- Difficulty paying attention.

CHAPTER 3:
Are There Different Grades of Severity of Concussions?

Uncertainty of an injury requires the input of a medical professional.

According to the following guidelines of the American Academy of Neurology (AAN), there are three grades of severity regarding concussions.

Grade 1 Concussion:
- Transient confusion; i.e. dazed or confused.
- No loss of consciousness but moderate to severe headache.
- Rapid recovery in which concussion symptoms abate in less than 15 minutes.

Grade 2 Concussion:
- The same as Grade 1 (short-term confusion and no loss of consciousness), but the concussion symptoms or cognitive abnormalities last longer than 15 minutes.

Grade 3 Concussion:
- Brain concussions at this level are normally characterized by any loss of consciousness, either short-term (a few seconds) or long-term (one minute or more).

Many organizations are getting more deeply involved in the concussion problems. The Mayo clinic offers baseline testing as do many hospitals and independent companies. Daily we are discovering more and more about the best and safest ways to deal with the issue.

If you are the least bit uncertain as to the extent of the concussion, ALWAYS seek medical treatment as soon as possible.

If you suspect a concussion has occurred, follow the American Academy of Neurology suggested four step concussion action plan.

CHAPTER 4: What to Do if a Concussion Occurs

If you suspect that someone has a sports-related concussion, the AAN suggests a four-step concussion action plan.

Step 1:

Remove the athlete from play, even if he or she says they can continue. Look for signs and symptoms of a concussion if your athlete has experienced a bump or a blow to the head or body. When in doubt, keep the athlete out of play. Understand that many athletes want to return to the game and will say anything to get back in the game. Do not use smelling salts or inhaled stimulants in that they may mask the symptoms.

Step 2:

The athlete should be evaluated by a healthcare professional with knowledge and experience in evaluating concussions and concussion symptoms. Parents, coaches, or spectators should not attempt to evaluate the severity of the head injury unless they are certified to do so. If no healthcare professionals are immediately available, you may perform an initial concussion assessment, which is detailed in Chapter 12.

Step 3:

Promptly inform the athlete's parents or guardians about the possible concussion, and tell them to consult with a healthcare professional experienced in evaluating concussions.

Step 4:

Keep the athlete out of play on the day of the injury and until a health care professional, experienced in evaluating concussions, says he or she is symptom-free and has released him or her to return to play. A repeat concussion that occurs before the brain recovers from the first, usually within a short period of time (hours, days, or weeks), can slow recovery or increase the likelihood of having long-term complications. ONLY allow the athlete to return to active practice or games AFTER the health care professional has granted him or her permission to do so.

A word of caution: Some experts feel, TOO MUCH inactivity after a concussion can be very detrimental. Watch the symptoms closely but don't overdo the activity. Allow the injured party to advance through the steps by supporting him or her and encourage them with assurances that they will be back with their friends and teammates soon.

CHAPTER 5: Aftercare of a Concussion

Learn the symptoms and be aware of changes from the norm, but don't be over-reactive.

Protocols for parents, family, and guardians

If your child has suffered a concussion, first watch for any of these signs:

- Appears confused or disoriented
- Is uncertain with regard to assignments or plays
- Is unsure of game, score, or opponent
- Moves awkwardly
- Responds slowly to questions
- Loses consciousness (even briefly)
- Displays mood swings or abnormal behavior patterns
- Limited memory of events before or after impact

It is important to listen to what your child is saying. Often, children will explain their symptoms or provide the opportunity to show their symptoms while being asked to describe if they feel hurt (where and how bad), what they are thinking about, how they feel (emotionally), and what their energy level may be. There are certain things that should be observed in the post-concussion period in order to determine whether or not symptoms are persisting for hours, days, or weeks. Much is dependent upon specifics, such as age, gender, normal behavior and activity level, any previous concussion history, etc. Every concussion is unique to the individual and recovery protocols must keep that in mind. One person may manifest little or no symptoms, while another experiences an array of symptoms. While some young athletes do not feel a disruption in their lives after having sustained a concussion, many find that their ability to effectively perform academic and other lifestyle activities (e.g., driving a car) is greatly affected by a concussive incident. In any case, lingering problems following a concussion are a signal that you should consult with a healthcare professional who is properly trained in concussion management. As with most medical problems, early detection and treatment of concussion is the best course of action in regard to recovery and prevention of future problems.

Protocols for coaches and trainers

- Number one: Do NOT rush the player back into play after he or she has exhibited concussion symptoms, even if the individual is your top performer. Aside from all the liability issues, it is simply wrong to do so. The parents have given you an amazing opportunity to coach their son or daughter and expect that your primary concern is the well-being of their child, no matter the child's age. As coaches, we are afforded huge responsibilities in our chosen endeavor. We must make certain that we are worthy of shouldering those responsibilities. The health and protection of that child is paramount.

- Stay in touch with the parents and check on the athlete's progress; support them in the aftercare protocols even when the player is begging you to "put me in Coach; I'm ready to play..."
- Check with teachers and administrators to make sure everyone is on the same page.
- Be a source of encouragement not only to the player, but also to the parents and other caregivers.
- Continue to assess your role in the recovery process knowing that you are an integral part of any decision for him or her to rejoin his or her team and teammates.

A word to medical professionals

- You are the most important decision maker in this whole process.
- The player cannot return to play without a written clearance from you.
- In sports, many times parents, friends, and coaches can exert pressure on medical professionals by saying things like, "Doc, I know my player, he's OK. Let me put him back in." Or, "Doc, I know my kid. He's going to be fine. He's ready to go. Trust me." Regardless of other people's advice, you make the final decision based upon your superior training and professionalism.
- If you are not a "sideline" doctor or medical tech and the player comes to your office for treatment, the coach and the parents trust you to make the right decision. Unfortunately, a word of caution is necessary. Not often, but sometimes, a medical professional does not like a given sport and can encourage parents and children to stay away from that sport because it is too dangerous or risky. After coaching for more than 35 years and having all my children participate in many different sports, I can honestly say that with the right equipment, coaching, conditioning, diet, and care, sports can be one of the greatest adventures a person can experience. The joy of camaraderie, the winning and losing together, and the opportunity to grow physically, emotionally, spiritually, and intellectually together with your peers are things from which no young person should be deprived. We hope that you are part of the encouraging process that is so appreciated by everyone concerned, and we applaud your dedication.

CHAPTER 6:
Professional's Protocols for Concussion Management

Tailor treatment to the individual. Everyone responds differently to a concussion.

- Often, the management of a concussion basically consists of requiring the individual to rest and, to a degree, limit physical exertion. This point also holds true for the thought processes and cognitive exertion.
- It is advisable to completely abstain from certain activities that require excessive brain stimulation, e.g. texting, spending too much time on the computer, listening to loud music, playing video games, etc.

Sports Concussion Institute (SCI), a very well respected authority in the area of athletic concussions, suggests four primary steps in concussion management:

1. Concussion education and awareness

2. Baseline concussion testing

3. Comprehensive neuropsychological clinical care

4. Review the STEPS covered in Chapter 4.

People react differently to concussions, so an individualized, gradual approach for the injured person to return them to athletics and academics is important. The point is to make certain we are returning a healthy and injury-free individual to his normal activities, both sports and academics.

Always err on the side of safety.

CHAPTER 7:
When to Seek Medical Attention after Receiving a Head Injury

Seek medical attention if the individual manifests any of the following symptoms after receiving a head injury:

- Headaches that worsen
- Changes in behavior
- Weakness or numbness in arms or legs
- Difficulty wakening
- Excessive vomiting
- Oral secretions of blood or fluids
- Changes in state of consciousness
- Difficulty recognizing people, places, names
- Increased confusion or irritability
- Speech problems: stuttering, slurring, mispronouncing words
- Seizures

It is vitally important to understand that it is never wrong to err on the side of safety. If a medical professional is available at the time of the injury, always defer to his or her expertise. Many sports require the presence of a medical professional at their games but not necessarily at the practices. Therefore, always have the phone number of the nearest team doctor or EMT for quick reference. Additionally, many concussions occur by accident during non-sports activities, such as playing, falling, car accidents, or simply life itself. So to be on the safe side, keep that phone number handy in case of an emergency.

CHAPTER 8: Protocols for Returning to Play or Activity

Return to play is a gradual, measured process.

There are four main steps to recovery

Step 1:
- Complete physical and cognitive rest until medical clearance
- No school attendance
- Strict limits on technology usage

Step 2:
- Return to school with modified involvement
- Continue limits on technology usage
- No heavy backpacks
- No tests, band, PE, or chorus
- Monitor symptoms
- Rest at home

Step 3:
- Continue academic limitations
- Attend school full time if possible
- Increase workload and homework
- Monitor symptoms
- Moderate rest at home but gradually increase activities

Step 4:
- Full recovery to academics
- Attend school full time
- Return to normal school schedules, tests, homework
- Resume normal activities, including sports

Scheduling recovery

Proceed from Step 1 to Step 2 only if the individual is symptom free for 24 hours. Continue to each subsequent step ONLY if the individual remains symptom free for 24 hours. If the individual is not symptom free at any level, remain at that level until he or she is symptom free.

What to watch for in the days and weeks following a concussion

The amount of time typically required for recovery from a traumatic brain injury can range from hours to a few days and, in some cases, even weeks depending upon gender, age, activity level, concussion history, and other personal factors. Every person's brain and injury situation is unique, and recovery must be tailored to the needs of the individual. While some athletes do not feel a disruption in their lives after having a concussion, many find difficulties in their ability to perform academically as well as in other daily activities, such as driving a car. In any case, lingering problems following a concussion should be a signal to consult with a healthcare professional who is properly trained in concussion management. As with most medical problems, early detection and treatment is the best course of action regarding recovery and prevention of future problems. Watch for changes in behavior, such as mood swings and outbursts of temper; activities that once brought pleasure may now become bothersome or be rejected entirely. Early in the healing process, it is important to reduce or eliminate as long as necessary activities such as texting, computer games, technical preoccupation, and even listening to loud music, all of which can retard the healing process and even cause unforeseen damage.

CHAPTER 9: Concussion Myths and Facts

Getting Educated.

Myth: You should not go to sleep after a concussion.

Fact: If current symptoms are being observed, they do not worsen, and new symptoms do not present themselves during the first minutes or hours immediately following a concussion, the standard recommendation is that if the injured person needs to sleep, he or she should do just that. Sleep is one of the most important processes the brain needs to begin the healing process. However, if you observe any new symptoms or if the existing ones appear to get worse, it is recommended that you seek emergency medical attention right away.

Myth: Any healthcare professional can treat a concussion.

Fact: Not always true. It is important that your medical professional is comfortable treating concussions and/or head, neck, and spinal issues. For more severe injuries of this sort, a more highly trained professional may be required—sometimes the specialized training offered by neurologists or neuropsychologists.

Myth: The injured party is usually aware of the extent of the injury.

Fact: Athletes often do not know when they have received a concussion. Athletes will not always admit or acknowledge that they have sustained a concussion. Consciously, athletes may downplay their symptoms, minimizing the severity of the injury, and/or attempt to play through the pain. They want to play, and sometimes that personal diagnosis may be the worst decision they can make. Often this self-diagnosis is supported by the parents, who want their child to play, or by the coach who holds the player in high regard and sees the loss of the player as placing his team in jeopardy of losing the game. If we are to consider ourselves responsible adults, we MUST consider what is best for the player and not act to satisfy any personal adult gratification.

Myth: You have to receive a blow to the head to receive a concussion.

Fact: Concussions can occur without hitting the head directly. For example, whiplash injuries can occur when an impact occurs to the body and the head or neck is suddenly jerked forward, backward, or side-to-side. The brain is accelerated in one direction, and then decelerated in another direction resulting in axonal shearing or tearing at the site of the injury. There are other concussion potentials when the body, not the head, is jarred or shaken severely.

Myth: It is safe to return to play if the symptoms are still present but less intense.

Fact: Experts from around the world agree that no athlete should be allowed to return to physical activity until he or she is totally asymptomatic (showing no symptoms). After a concussion, the brain needs rest and time to heal, and this cannot happen when it is subjected to physical activity (athletic or otherwise), cognitive exertion (classroom or even homework), and the emotional mood swings that often accompany an injury. All these play an important role in recognizing changing behavior patterns in a person's life. Returning a child or teenager to physical and cognitive activities before symptoms are resolved risks further injury, can decrease the athlete's performance level, and even potentially exacerbate debilitative long-term effects such as depression, anxiety, and in some cases, more chronic issues.

Myth: A concussion only affects the injured individual.

Fact: A concussion, just like any injury, can have profound effects on everyone in the athlete's circle of influence, including parents and family, coaches, academic personnel, and healthcare professionals. Having said that, it is vital to treat concussions from a multidisciplinary approach. Every athlete can manifest the results of a concussion in his or her own way.

Care should be taken to evaluate the recovery process and to educate one another on the symptoms, aftercare, and reentry of athletes into their schools and regular play activities as well as their sports. Understanding these myths and facts is necessary in order for us to elevate our care to meet the responsibilities placed upon us.

CHAPTER 10:
How Do We Prevent or Reduce the Incidences of Concussions?

Anyone can get a concussion, in or out of sports, but prevention is a by-product of education.

Team sports present a variable approach to the issue. Any sport that requires a helmet is the first to be considered. But according to helmet manufactures and the National Operating Committee on Standards for Athletic Equipment (NOCSAE), a helmet is designed to protect against skull fractures, not to prevent concussions. It goes without saying that helmets in certain sports are absolutely necessary and probably do reduce instances of concussion, but due to the legal climate, the manufactures are inhibited from using words like: "prevention, reducing, lowers," etc., for fear of the other word..."lawsuit."

1. **Football:**

    The issues are fairly comprehensive.

    - It begins with the manufacturer of the helmet. The NOCSAE is the official tester of helmets from the youth level through the professional. After initial testing, most organizations require reconditioning of helmets every two years. The helmets are sent to a reconditioning company operating under NOCSAE standards, which puts them through a series of tests to determine whether or not they are safe. If the helmets are determined to be unsafe, they are removed from service. If the helmets are deemed "safe," interior helmet pads and hardware are replaced, and the helmets are returned to the organization.

    - The accountability for keeping the helmets safe after they have been approved becomes the responsibility of the local organization. They should have an equipment manager working with the various teams. The equipment manager should be required to attend specific classes designed to help him understand the helmet specifics. Get information about the availability of these classes by contacting NOCSAE or the local high school coach.

    - Make certain all the hardware (screws, clamps, etc.) is installed properly.

    - Be careful that helmet snaps are snug, but not overly tight. Tightening the snaps too much can cause tiny fractures on the helmet snap points, thus negating the protective value of the helmet. These helmets are expensive, so make sure the equipment personnel understand their jobs.

    - Constant evaluation of the helmet is part of the process. Even the wrong kind of paint can cause a helmet to fail, so only use the paint or sealer recommended by the manufacturer.

    - One of the most important issues is making absolutely certain the helmet fits properly. When the athlete puts the helmet on, the fit should be carefully checked. A helmet that is too loose could lead to a potential concussion. One that is too tight will cause headaches. Fitting the helmet to make sure it is snug all around the head is vital. It takes a little extra time to get it right, but this kind of attention will maximize prevention protocols.

- Listen to the athlete. He or she will tell you if it is comfortable. Also, that comfort level may change during the season. The fit can change radically at considerable altitude changes. AND, kids grow. They get bigger and so do their heads. (Sometimes the coach's head gets bigger too, but that's a different story.)
- The chinstrap is also important. Most of the players are not pros and are not trying to make a style statement by not wearing a chinstrap or leaving it undone. Not wearing a chinstrap is a penalty at most levels. The chinstrap should be snug but not too tight.
- In addition to a huge variety of facemasks, an important attachment to the helmet is the mouthpiece. Many organizations have a standard approved mouthpiece that can be adequate, but for athletes with braces or jaw problems, it's better to have a dentist or an orthodontist approve the mouthpiece. One more thing about mouthpieces: most are designed to go over the upper teeth, but research is showing that a mouthpiece that protects both the upper and lower jaw can have very positive results. Most youth level rules require that the mouthpiece attach to the facemask, and it is usually a one-piece rubber or vulcanized apparatus.

2. Hockey:

Next in line, with a light Kevlar helmet that may or may not have a visor or even a cage.

- Again, the manufacturer is vitally important. We recommend an approved, certified helmet that has stood the test of time. There are bad helmets out there, and price cannot be the determining factor in trying to prevent or reduce instances of concussion.
- The same rules that apply to football helmets and mouthpieces apply to hockey as well. The greatest difference is in the chinstrap. Half the players either do not buckle up the chinstrap or they do not have one. This is not a good policy for obvious reasons.

3. Cycling:

Particularly competitive cycling, has a lot of collisions, many at very high speeds. The cycling helmet is very different.

- It is designed for protection but also must be aerodynamic to afford the cyclist the least possible wind resistance.
- Again, the manufacturer is the key. Take the time to check out the helmet manufacturer, design, and road-tested results. How do they compare with other suppliers in the area of concussions?

4. Baseball:

Also has instances of concussion. The greatest fear most youngsters have is being hit by a pitch thrown from the mound. However, far more injuries occur in baseball by sliding into a base, running into another player, or two or more players trying to make a play in the field. Batters wear a helmet; fielders do not. In baseball, one of the great preventions of injury comes from proper field communication. The best coaches spend time with the players going over verbal signals and on field calls.

5. Boxing and mixed martial arts:

Presents the most serious potential for injury. After all, the object and supreme success of the sport is to render the opponent unconscious, which is the definition of a concussion. Some of the greatest boxers in the long, colorful history of the sport have suffered from catastrophic injuries after they have left the sport. We used to call them "punch-drunk" or "palookas," because they were either incoherent in interviews or stuttered so badly that others had difficulty understanding them. Some have acquired diseases like Parkinson's or ALS or have been institutionalized because of beatings they took in the ring. Others have died from the punishment they absorbed during the course of a fight. Boxing is an institution in many countries around the world, and it does not seem likely that it will change.

Sports that do not require a helmet

1. **Soccer:**

    Research is revealing that more soccer players are experiencing concussions. One of the primary issues is the idea of wearing a helmet or not. In most programs at any level, helmets are not required. But is that a good thing? The purists believe that helmets are unnecessary, since soccer is a "non-contact" sport. The 2014 World Cup would suggest otherwise. Some believe that a helmet would destroy the aesthetics or the purity of the sport. What about the safety of the athlete? Here's an interesting fact: women soccer players have greater incidences of concussions than men. What is more disturbing is that many teachers and researchers are reporting noticeable memory issues in young soccer players, particularly from "heading" the ball. It might be time to rethink the issue of helmets in soccer. The speed of the ball can be extreme and could be dangerous if a player attempts to radically change the flight of the ball with his or her head.

2. **Cheerleading:**

    The most recent studies rank cheerleading close to the top in instances of concussion. Various stunts, many of them previously unacceptable due to the risk factors, have been included. Competition in cheerleading is amazing—local, regional, state, even nationwide events pit cheerleading teams against each other in a variety of levels and styles. Many of the most successful organizations send their cheerleaders to private cheer camps operated by professional coaches. Many of these camps are extremely expensive in addition to the various uniforms, kick pants, gloves, shoes, etc. The problem is that many organizations have a more intense focus on winning these events than on what is best for their cheerleaders. I believe that cheerleading is great. The support and encouragement that these young people bring to their athletic teams is absolutely commendable. However, the safety issues need to be addressed. The throws and complexity of some of the routines are amazing, but the risk factor must be emphasized not only to the young participants, but also to the parents AND their coaches, professional or amateur.

3. **Other Sports:**

    There are many other sports, such as basketball, skateboarding, lacrosse, wrestling, rugby, BMX cycling, kids rodeo, waterpolo and gymnastics, which also need to be addressed; however, it must be remembered that a concussion can occur at play, at work, at school, or anywhere people are going to be active and involved.

Getting Involved.

CHAPTER 11:
Can We Prevent Concussions From Ever Happening?

Absolutely not! Can we reduce the incidences? Absolutely yes! How? Many parents ask, "How can we get involved with our athlete?" The following suggestions are a few ways to do just that.

- **Stay abreast with the research and changes in equipment.** There are many people doing great work in trying to forge equipment that protects the athlete. On the horizon are a number of products that are able to "sense" the potential of a concussion via certain devices that attach to a helmet or headband.
- **Know the rules of the game.** If there are questionable issues, change them.
- **Get involved with the organization**—if not in coaching, then in board positions. These organizations do not function without honest, dedicated administrators who toil behind the scenes for little or no acclaim, and they are always looking for good folks to pitch in and make it all work.
- **Get to know your coach.** Make sure the coaches know what they are doing. Most coaches are great people and dedicated to their sport. But occasionally, the motivation for coaching, particularly at the youth levels, is suspect. I've heard coaches say, "I'm in it for the kids." What they mean is, "I'm in it for MY kid." They are focused on living vicariously through the victories of their children rather than on team endeavors. To the devoted coaches: YOU are the best! Your dedication, selfless sacrifices, and willingness to be there for the kids are virtues that should be praised and respected. The negative things to which I allude are not directed at you, the real coaches, but at a very few who take our sport and make it all about them. If you want to be called "coach" (a profound title), be worthy. Take the classes, go to clinics, and get educated. Understand that as a coach, you are a teacher, a leader, a counselor, a guide, and in many cases, a hero to some young person who needs all that and more. It has been said, "I'm only one person, and how can I change the world?" Yet as a coach, you will discover that you may be the world to one young person. Coaching is a calling. Winning is a by-product of everything you do. It starts with honor, integrity, ethics, sportsmanship, character, scholastics, good citizenship, and every good "ism" you can think of. Do not compromise your ethics for some on-field victory that is gained by bending the rules, cheating, or putting your players at risk.

- **Be supportive, not negative.** Too often teams and organizations fall apart because a couple of folks who do not like the way things are going, and rather than being constructive, they become the official team critics; they cause dissention among other parents by tearing down the coaches behind their backs and undermining anything with which they do not agree. Learn from these folks and do the opposite.
- **Coach training:** Since coaches are required to learn CPR and First Aid, we need to offer certification training for concussion awareness and protocols. Some hospitals and clinics offer classes, but much more needs to be done to help coaches with certification.

The Do's and Don'ts of On-field Assessment.

CHAPTER 12:
The On-Field Assessment Guide (THE CARD)

Don'ts
- Don't remove the player's helmet until a comprehensive assessment is made. If the player is suffering from head, neck, or spinal trauma, removing the helmet could cause dangerous consequences.
- Don't try to help the player up into a sitting or standing position until the assessment has been completed.
- Don't allow a crowd around the injured player, especially other players, fans, or parents. Often the concern parents show may cause the player to panic or react negatively.

Do's
- When first approaching the injured player, keep him or her calm and motionless. Make sure YOU are under control.
- Determine whether or not the player is conscious. If not, immediately contact emergency services (911). There should also be a contact number for a local emergency facility in the event the 911 number is busy or slow.
- If the player is awake, now is the time for communication. It is known as the "One second response". Ask basic questions beginning with, "Where does it hurt?" This is your first opportunity to begin assessing the injury. Ask the injured athlete to describe the impact. Is the speech slurred or labored? Can the player respond in a reasonable length of time to questions concerning the day, the time, the opponent, etc? Check the "symptoms information section" (Chapter 2) in this workbook to determine whether or not the player needs to be transported or if it is an injury that can be addressed on the field.
- Absolutely no smelling salts or stimulants that cause a startled response.
- Certain tests can be revealing. Have the player stick out his tongue and move it to the left, right, up, and down. Sounds silly, but it can be very helpful. Have the player move his or her eyes by following your finger. Also, see how quickly the pupils respond to light or the absence of light. In other words, are the pupils dilating or pinpointing? At night, the field lights are adequate. During the day, sunlight or a bright sky is good.
- If the player is reacting positively, ask him or her if he would like to sit up. Be very patient at this point. Reassure the player with a statement such as, "Right now, you're the only one we are thinking about, so take all the time you need."

- Ask the player to remove his or her helmet only if the assessment has been positive. Do NOT help him or her take the helmet off. Let him or her do it on his or her own. Watch the player's facial expressions very carefully and keep the communication going. Keep asking for the player's input on any other potential injuries, but the main focus should be on the head, neck, and spinal areas.

- If possible, have the player walk off the field slowly, only helping if it is needed.

- Do NOT leave the injured player unattended on the sideline.

- Before a return to play, your field doctor or medical professional MUST clear the athlete. If you or your staff is not certified for on-field injury assessment, the ONLY decision is that the athlete does not return to play until a professional has assessed him or her. And if no one on your staff is qualified, my question is, "Why not?" There are plenty of classes offered by local hospitals, your high school coaching staff, and coaching clinics whose curriculum includes American Red Cross First Aid, CPR instruction, and head trauma instruction. Remember, you're a coach. So be the best one you can be, and that means getting educated on more than just running plays or having a great defense. It also means you are a professional. Your integrity, character, and ethics are on display every practice and every game. Do not compromise. Be firm but fair. Unfortunately we are living in a very litigious society, and if you do not want to distressfully appear in court some day, get certified* and support the rules of on-field care.

Remember, any effective concussion management begins well before the injury actually occurs. It starts with properly educating athletes, parents, coaches, athletic trainers, teachers, and other people in the athlete's life. Not only does this allow the dispersal of new, cutting-edge information directed to people involved in youth sports, but it also provides a forum for questions to be answered by leaders in the field of concussion management.

It is necessary for sports organizations to create and establish a given set of standards in order to offer certification training for concussion awareness and protocols. Some hospitals and clinics offer classes, but much more needs to be done to help coaches with certification. We can help.

Concussion Awareness: Coach Certification Program

Certification regarding head trauma is essential for coaches, trainers, managers, etc., regardless of sport venue.

CERTIFICATION WILL INCLUDE:

- On-line test
- Resource guide (download or printed copy
- Certification of Completion
- Continuing Education Units (CEU)
- May include Audio or video DVD

Visit our website for information and start date for Concussion Awareness Certification program. **ConcussionAwarenessInstitute.com**

Or scan the QR code to the right with your smartphone

Research and Development.

CHAPTER 13:
What is Being Done to Research the Long- and Short-Term Issues and Damages Caused by Concussions?

If you research the Internet, you will find literally millions of websites with the word "concussion" in their lead pages. More than ninety-five percent of these websites are trying to sell you something. Don't get me wrong; some of the things they are trying to sell you may have value, but you really have to search a long time before you find one.

However, the greatest problem is that there is little known about concussions. The effects of a concussion to the brain, the symptoms, the recovery from concussion, and the return to play are all issues which need to be addressed and we do so in several chapters in this book. There is a great deal of research regarding the development of better equipment, testing systems, and simply a deeper understanding of the concussion itself. We would like guarantees and promises. However, because of our "lawsuit happy" society and an abundance of lawyers who have to make a living, no one wants to use words like "cure," "reduction," "better," and so on. The sports equipment manufacturers know that if someone is using their equipment and gets injured, unless they have surrounded their labels with disclaimer language, they are wide open to serious risk management suits. I think Shakespeare wrote something about lawyers, and then the Eagles amped it up a bit.

Very soon, the market will be inundated with "Sensor" products that actually measure the degree of impact the body experiences when a collision occurs. The NFL may mandate a product for the 2015 season, but don't get too excited, because the cost is absolutely prohibitive for anyone except the NFL. There are varying products soon to be available with pricing ranging from $89.00 up to several hundred dollars. A company called "Heads Up" Impact Sensor will be making a really superior product available for under $50.00, which should appeal to the youth market. This product is available not only for helmeted sports, but for non-helmeted sports as well. Most products will report to a computer or cell phone, which will require someone to watch the computer or cell phone at all times. The Heads Up product does not need a secondary reporting system in that when the impact exceeds a certain "g" force level, a light system alerts anyone in the vicinity that a potential injury has just occurred.

CHAPTER 14: A Word to Coaches

Don't compromise your integrity, character or ethics.

Having coached for more than 35 years...

The panorama of sports has changed radically. In the early years of my coaching experience, we used to show up on the first day of practice and there were so many kids, we had to beat them off with a stick, figuratively speaking. This is no longer the case. Today, you have to recruit heavily at the youth level and be involved with everything, including fundraising, (from candy sales to really creative stuff, such as Vegas nights and carnivals) getting flyers into schools, car rallies, and so much more. Oh, by the way, you also have to coach. When I was coaching high school and youth football at the same time, my wife wanted to know what I was doing for a living. All the youth involvement was non-paid volunteer work. High school coaching paid a stipend. After counting the hours one year and the money we made, it worked out to a little less than 11 cents an hour. Sounds funny, but ask the high school assistant coaches. Today, the kids in schools are trying to emulate the pro athletes; they spend so much of their life playing video games, it's unbelievable. It used to be that the parents wanted the kids out of the house playing because they knew it was healthy and would get the kids away from television. One of the broadest changes over the years has to do with parents' attitudes. I spoke earlier about the positive involvement parents can have, but it seems that many folks now see television and video games as a fantastic baby sitter, one that not only entertains the kids but also keeps them out of Mom and Dad's hair.

Let's talk about coaching ethics

This information applies to coaches regardless of the sport they coach. I also encourage teachers, administrators, and medical professionals as well as parents to read this and gain a little more insight into the issues that coaches face every day.

The philosophy of the ethical coach

To promote, refine, and incorporate excellence in the high calling of coaching for the betterment and growth of youngsters and young men and women; to teach, encourage, and invest in these athletes; to be role models of honesty and ethics in the arena of competition; to set aside any personal gain or visions of glory by placing the needs of those athletes in front of our own.

Alfred Baden Powell, founder of the Boys Scouts, stated, "Never has a man stood as tall as when he has stooped to help a child." In youth football, coaches for years have been instructed to set aside "adult lust for glory" and replace it with the elevation of our youth to the joy of positive self-esteem and confidence. All youth, high schools, and colleges, along with their coaches, should be the flag bearers of ethics, integrity, and honor for every community in which we have the privilege of coaching.

Coaching Objectives

- Make this game that we love more than just a great experience for kids, but also for the parents, grandparents, and friends of the players.

- Teach winning as a "by-product" of scholastics, sportsmanship, citizenship, obedience, discipline, and integrity. There are many life principles that can be taught through sports.

- Understand and teach that sports are GAMES! It is neither the beginning nor the end of life. The sun WILL come up tomorrow.

- Learn and equip ourselves with the tools necessary to translate the language of our craft into a language that can be understood and applied by youngsters. Be a student of the game as well as a coach.

- Learn to build a forum for coaches that will break down walls that exist between individuals and local organizations. Form a fellowship of coaches who sincerely want to be better, more productive, and feel good about the things they are bringing to the coaching ranks.

- Learn how to not only coach but also share your knowledge with other less experienced coaches in order that the very foundation of coaching will be elevated.

- Make a commitment, not an excuse, to be part of a body whose desire is to raise the standards of coaching at every level.

- Winning is important but not at all costs. To win through honest effort with uncompromising integrity is a joy. To win at the expense of ethics is a hollow victory indeed.

- When the season is over, what will your player say about you? Hopefully, that player has had a positive educational experience filled with not only plays and memories but also with life-lessons that will have a constructive effect on their future. I have made some wonderful lifelong friendships with parents and players alike, relationships that have changed MY life in so many ways. I feel immense gratitude toward my players and I hope they feel the same toward me.

EXPECTATIONS:

What can we expect out of a coach? First of all, communication. We can set aside the barriers that exist between team rivalries, teachers, administrators, parents and fans. AND between coaches in order to learn who we are as individuals. Often there are histories of feuds and differences between coaches not only from competing cities, but within that same city... and without communication, these differences can turn into wars!.. Sometimes the reasons for the feuds are long forgotten, but the feud continues "just because that's the way it is!!!" So often when people have the opportunity to meet face to face and discuss the things important to them as individuals, we find that we are not all that different from each other. Sometimes there are comments made which are taken out of context and even misquoted to others. These comments are then blown out of proportion and become a source and a reason to start a war, but if they were taken IN context and directly to the parties involved, the problem would never even manifest itself.

Coaches can meet for fellowship, camaraderie, and even for instruction. We are more familiar with the problems and limitations in coaching athletes than anyone. Often when a youth coach and a high school coach in the same community don't communicate, problems occur. It's difficult for a high school coach to understand the limitations of a 2 hour practice 3 times a week, when he is running 2-a- days or films during lunch period and early outs for specialists! Why not pool information, instead of pooling ignorance? Don't misunderstand me, ignorance is simply lack of knowledge in a specific area. We can conduct our own internal sessions on everything from staff organization to position coaching; from scouting to special teams. We can even schedule off-season activities, get-togethers, break bread together (eating.... which is one of my personal favorites). We can develop coaching protocols for new coaches, document the experiences of the older coaches; become a source of ideas, a kind of think tank for coaches. We can even expand eventually to inculcate other coaches from other organizations. We as coaches can form an organization like this, and unquestionably, it will fill a vacuum.

There are a couple of more items that I would like to address:

1. Chain of Command: Whenever possible we would like to keep problems within team confines, but sometimes it's necessary to exercise a chain of command. In issues of coaching, each organization has their own Coach's rep or athletic director. It's our job to discuss situations that need outside involvement. If a coach cannot get any satisfaction from his city's coach's rep, that coach can come up the chain of command to the athletic director then to the administrator and thereby follow the necessary steps to get these things resolved.

2. I want to talk for a minute about Rule Changes. So often during the year I hear coaches come up with a great idea for a rule change or a suggestion that will make things work better. Then nothing happens. We need to write these ideas down, get them to the head coach then the athletic director. Get together with the referee's reps, dissect the ideas, if appropriate, articulate them in writing and present them to the Governing Body for your sport for consideration at the appropriate time.

Lastly THE REALITY:

Every one of us knows that there are some coaches out there that will do ANYTHING to win; whether it's lying, falsifying documents, cheating in a thousand different ways, illegal recruiting, abusing the system and my God why do we just sit back and watch it happen? Winston Churchill made one of the most profound statements in history in 1939 when Hitler was initiating the holocaust and the genocide of the Jews. He said, (quoting John Locke) "The only thing necessary for evil to abound, is for good people to sit back and do nothing!" It's time to make a stand for the ethics of coaching. If something bad is going on and you know it, you're not a 'rat' if you report it. You're simply doing the RIGHT thing. So often the kids are the ones who pay a heavy price for some adult who just can't seem to conduct himself honorably and honestly.

SUMMARY:

We have an opportunity to be the kind of coaches that will have a tremendous impact upon our organizations for years to come if we have enough people who are willing to not only take a stand, but to make a commitment. There are three kinds of people who are engaged in coaching... 1. Those that make it happen, 2. those that watch it happen, and 3. those that don't know WHAT happened. There is no need to suffer from the "Paralysis of Analysis". Make a commitment NOW. Be a part of the solution not a part of the problem.

The Sports Concussion Analytical Tool and Baseline Testing.

CHAPTER 15:
What Is The Issue of "Baseline Testing?"

I would like to thank Mr. Lance Townend of Canadian Sports Risk Management, for his kindness in allowing us to reprint some of the information his company developed in the area of baseline testing:

> One of the most significant discoveries of the Geneva Conference when the Sports Concussion Analytical Tool was developed was the determination that a Baseline was needed as a means of comparison when a SCAT test was administered. With the baseline, conclusive results could now be obtained.

The SCAT (Sports Concussion Analytical Test) and SCAT2 tests were developed by the Geneva Medical Convention in Switzerland when doctors from all over the world met to discuss concussions, specifically concerning testing, diagnosis and treatments. Their resultant publication of the SCAT & SCAT2 tests have been accepted throughout amateur and professional sports groups and associations.

With the invention of the SCAT2 and Baseline Measurement, it is possible to get a very accurate difference between pre and post incident. The problem with getting the Baseline measurement has always been the most difficult part of Concussion Treatment due to the issue of getting athletes to complete a baseline test at the beginning of a season. Then there is the issue of logistics. The sheer numbers of this process are mind boggling, not to mention the management of that information which will require man-power and computers capable of being organized to use that information, along with Medical Professionals that can interpret the data in order to help the athlete recover.

Using a narrator to eliminate questioning bias, the questions and instructions are completed online with visual aids and simple to follow instructions. All athletes, children, adolescents/teen, and adults are able to complete the tests on-line so that we obtain the all-important baseline score. All testing results are of course encrypted, confidential and secure.

The cost of Baseline testing varies considerably throughout the country. Many hospitals, for example any Mayo Clinic affiliate will offer a cost free program to various organizations. Other clinics and medical centers will offer testing for anywhere from $10.00 per individual to over $50.00, depending upon the depth of the testing. Start with local hospitals and go from there.

CHAPTER 16:
Case Studies

I would like to preface this chapter by reiterating that the vast majority of concussions are mild and do not develop into catastrophic conditions. However, it serves us well to let folks know that a concussion is still a serious issue. So, presented below are a couple of cases addressing the more serious injuries.

Case Study One - Dr. Stephanie Mills: 2014 Ms. America and mom.

A call from the school came in: "Your daughter was knocked out in gym class. Please pick her up immediately." Brooke was an "A" student as a freshman. That morning she bent down to pick up a ball as a boy kicked it. His foot, the ball, and her head all made simultaneous contact, and she blacked out. In the days after the accident, Brooke's headaches worsened. As a chiropractor, her mom was able to give her frequent spinal adjustments to ease her head pain and malaise, but her memory was an issue. Brooke would walk into a room and not remember why, she lost memories of family vacations, and she struggled to remember what was taught in her classes before her head trauma occurred. Brooke had suffered a concussion.

At first, Brooke committed herself to recovering with cognitive rest: no texting, no television, no school, or studying. Physical activities ceased, including her dance team. After a week of missed school and activities, the pressure to return became undeniable. Brooke had no baseline concussion testing prior to her trauma. Doctors had no way to prove to teachers and coaches whether she was ready to resume normal activities.

As a parent, Dr. Mills needed to become her daughter's advocate. When the guidance counselor suggested Brooke return to gym class just days after her impact, her mother refused. As a chiropractor, Dr. Mills knew the risk of Secondary Impact Syndrome. A second concussion before the first healed completely could be more devastating and possibly deadly. Brooke spent the remainder of her freshman year struggling in school. As of this printing, many of her memories still have not returned. Protective gear in gym class may have helped her to avoid injury. Many concussions cannot be prevented, but the best solution is to institute baseline testing for all middle and high school students. The chance of missing a concussion diagnosis is greatly reduced and allows better monitoring of the recovery process.

Case Study Two - Mike Shaw   (The Author)

I was a fullback in high school and, upon occasion, carried the football. In one game I apparently had a good run up the middle and was tackled. My helmet was a single bar suspension helmet (these are not used anymore). When I went down, my facemask hit the ground, and the helmet flew off. The safety, who may have been auditioning to be the punter kicked me square in my forehead. According to the witnesses, I jumped up and was pulled back into the huddle as the other guy was thrown out of the game. Our quarterback felt that the play was pretty good, so he called it again. My team formed up on the line of scrimmage, the center snapped the ball, the quarterback turned to hand it to me, but I wasn't there. I was back where the huddle was formed, staring into the sky. I'm told that I was taken off the field, went to the hospital, was released, and went home.

The game had been played on a Thursday evening. The next morning, I woke up and went to school with every intention of playing football that day. My coach saw me walking down the hall and asked me how I was doing. I said. "Great, we're going to whip Beal Tech today." He looked at me strangely and asked, "What day is it?" I said, "Thursday." He said, "OK, come with me." He put me in his car and drove me back to the hospital. I had completely lost 24 hours out of my life. I have no recollection of ever playing in that game. The memory is gone. I'm telling this from eyewitness accounts. I suffered severe headaches for a week, but after that, there were no issues at all. I was very blessed not to have any complications, but the memory loss was very disconcerting.

I have had several occasions that I described as having my "bell rung," not just from sports but from a car accident, falling down a flight of stairs, a window closing with force on the back of my head, and generally engaging in what insurance actuarial adjusters say are, "high risk activities." It's called LIFE! We can't go through life cloistered and protected from possible negative consequences that can fall on anyone. We can experience our lives with joy and delight, knowing that what lies ahead will be predicated on not the events themselves, but how we respond to them.

Coach and Author Michael (Mike) Shaw Bio

Mike was born in Canada. He has played competitive Hockey, Football, Basketball, Baseball, Volleyball, Track and Field, Swimming and Diving, Wrestling, Tennis, Badminton and more. He has always been close to sports. He worked for Sports Productions, Inc., Cleveland, Ohio then, started his own company in conjunction with the American Basketball Assn. He came to California in 1969, and married Toni. They raised three children, Casey, Stephanie and Cory. He coached football for 35 years at the youth level and high school. He coached youth football in Rowland Heights for 28 years as a head coach compiling a record of 286 wins and 33 losses, but more importantly, he and his staff won more sportsmanship and scholastic awards than any coaching staff in the country. For a number of years Mike has directed some of the finest coaching clinics in the nation. He has been the Vice President of the National Football Foundation and Hall of Fame, and is the 1st youth football coach to be named to the Hall of Fame.

Mike has worked with the United States Olympic Committee and has written other books for athletes. He is currently a Chaplain and owns two companies: Coaching Software Solutions, LLC and CSC Enterprises, LLC a real estate investment firm.

CHAPTER 17:
Using this Book as a Fundraiser

The book, "Concussion Awareness", can greatly enhance various groups particularly youth organizations, in necessary fundraising, because of the constant need money to pay for equipment, fields, officials, insurance and a host of other expenses.

Any successful fundraiser needs to express the following factors:

1. Who your organization is.
2. Why you need money.
3. The problem of concussions
4. How this book addresses the problem.
5. How the business you are approaching may participate.
6. Outline the gain for the business.

Following are a few examples:

Appeal to Local Businesses:

To Whom it may Concern:

I represent _____, a local _____ organization and we are asking for your help in dealing with a serious issue.

As you are probably aware, the problem of concussions has become a grave concern regardless of the sport. We feel it is vital for our organization to deal with the issue as broadly as possible. The book, "Concussion Awareness," has been made available to us at a deeply discounted price. This book deals with everything from explaining what a concussion is, the symptoms, the protocols in dealing with the injury, the aftercare and return to play. It has sections on the myths and facts of concussion, the advances in reducing such injuries, and the need to get this book into the hands of parents, coaches, trainers, administrators, teachers and even the players themselves. It is written in easy to understand language, but it can be of great value to even medical professionals.

Our cost is only $_____* per book. We would like to ask for your participation in that cost. In return for your cooperation, depending upon the amount you would be willing to invest, we would like to offer you advertising space in the book, and/or a mention on the public address system at our home games to express our gratitude for your co-sponsorship.

This book should be part of every sports organizations commitment to provide a safe andsecure environment for all participants. We would like to be able to give this book to every parent, coach, teacher, administrator, and player in our organization. We have a total of____ players,____ coaches,____ parents, and ____ teachers and administrators, for a total of _____ participants in our programs.

We would like to make an appointment to see you,show you the book and determine the level at which you would like to participate.

I'll contact you in the next few days. Thank you for your consideration in helping us deal withthis vitally important issue.

Signature _____

* Please go to our website ConcussionAwarenessInstitute.com for pricing information. For additional ideas on fundraising, please visit our website at:
ConcussionAwarenessInstitute.com

If your organization opts for an internal fundraiser, we suggest the following:

1. Determine how much money you need to pay for books for every player in your program.
2. Add $___ to your cost of registration to account for the number of books you need.
3. Add $___ to the cost to determine the actual profit per book you need to meet the goal of the fundraiser.
4. You can still get local merchants to participate by selling ad space in the book (certain minimums are required) or by printing an insert for the book, with various ads for these local merchants.

If your organization opts for a letter program to businesses, we suggest the following:

Direct mail with telephone follow-up.
Normally, a direct mail program will yield approximately a 1.5% return based on the number of letters you send. Considering the cost of postage, labor, transporting the mail to the post office, etc., and unless you have a completely voluntary program, the cost is high compared to the return. However, through various sources, we have discovered that this return can be tremendously enhanced by a follow up program over the phone. This kind of return can expect a 15 to 20% return, which is substantial and would certainly exceed any costs by a considerable amount. The telephone follow up is extremely important and should include many of the factors mentioned earlier:

1. Who are you? What organization is asking for the money. Be specific.
2. Explain why you need the money, or how it will be used?
3. What part the book will play in your fundraising program?
4. Some basic concerns related to concussions.
5. How the book addresses those concerns.
6. How the business your are approaching can participate and
7. What benefits they can derive through their participation.

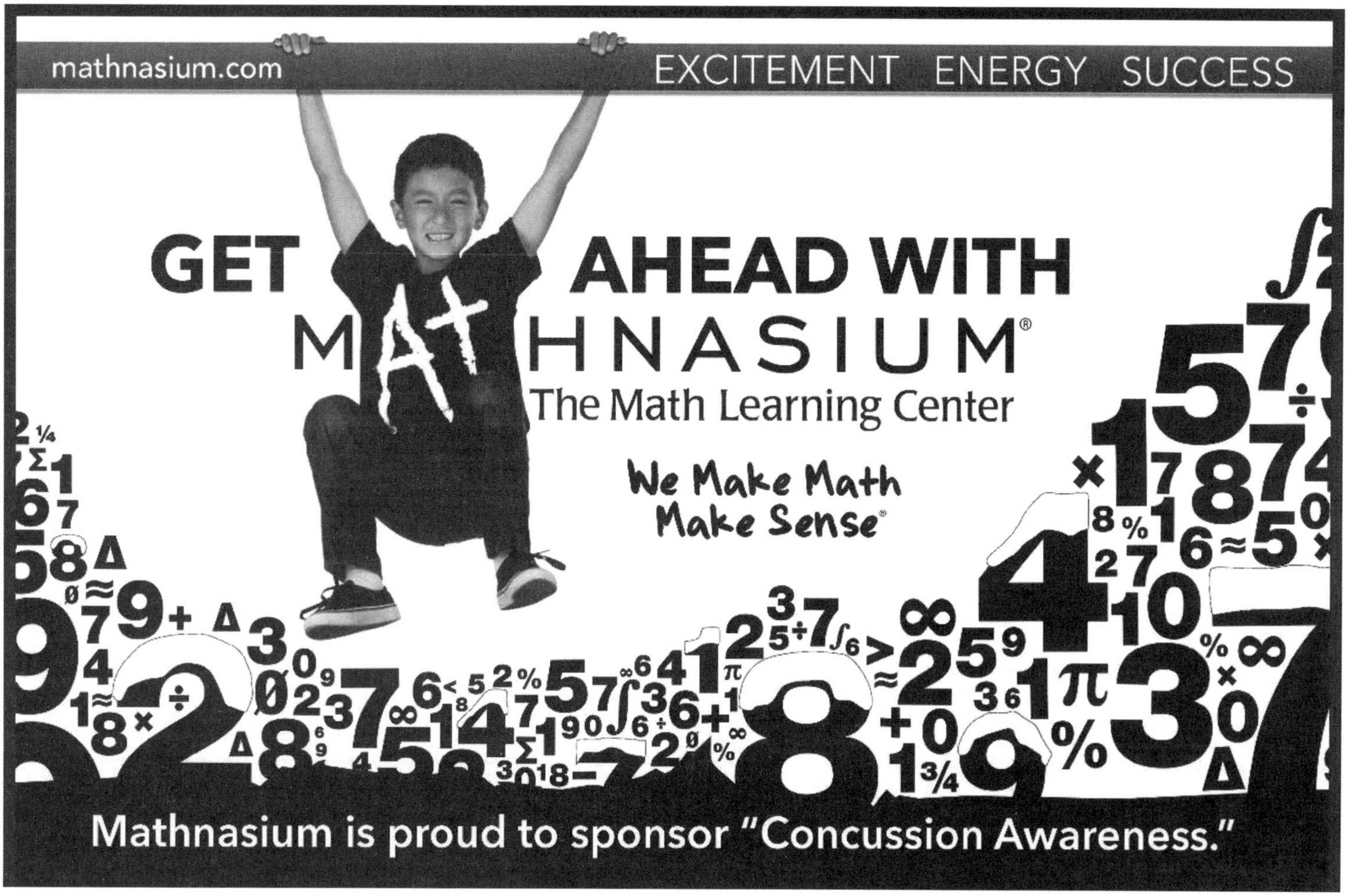

mathnasium.com   EXCITEMENT ENERGY SUCCESS

GET AHEAD WITH MATHNASIUM®
The Math Learning Center

We Make Math Make Sense®

Mathnasium is proud to sponsor "Concussion Awareness."

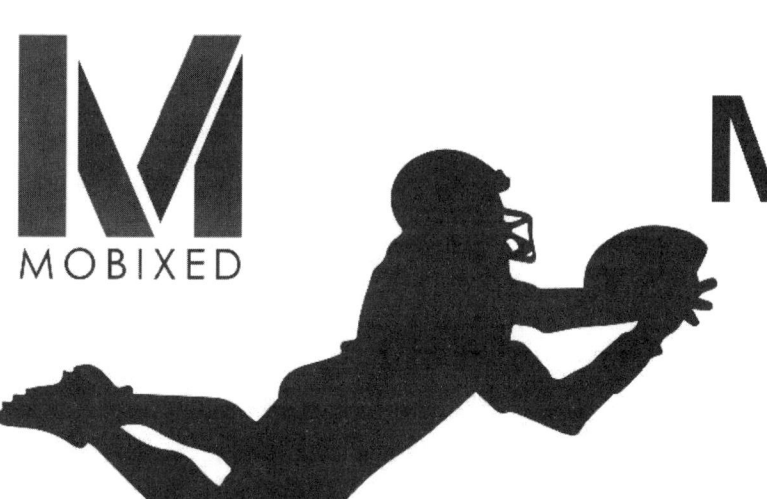

MOBIXED

MOBIXED

We support the "Concussion Awareness" book, athletes, parents and coaches – who make sports better for us all.

(949) 751-6109 • www.mobixed.com
iOS, Android, WIndows, Cordova PhoneGap